RENAL DIET COOKBOOK 2021

SECRETS OF KIDNEY DISEASE: CHALLENGE YOURSELF TO LIVING HEALTHIER IN 30 DAYS:

⭐⭐⭐

AM I SUITABLE FOR PERITONEAL DIALYSIS

KIDNEY CLEANSE AND ITS RECIPES

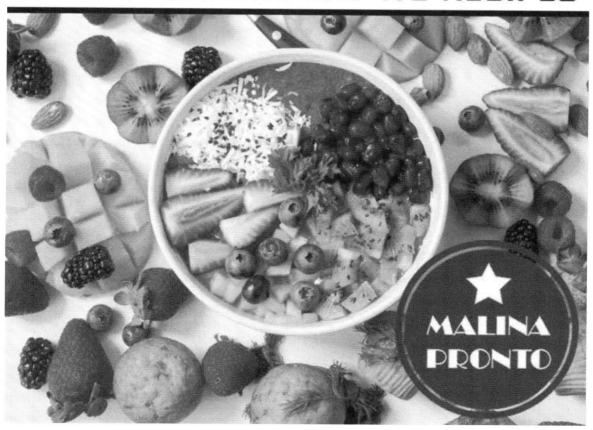

MALINA PRONTO

Renal Diet Cookbook 2021:
Secrets Of Kidney Disease:
Challenge Yourself To Living Healthier In 30 Days:
Am I Suitable For Peritoneal Dialysis:
Kidney Cleanse And Its Recipes

Renal Diet

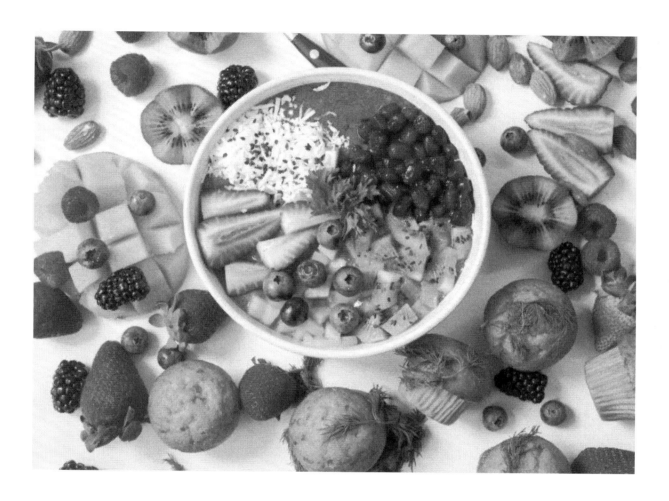

A Renal eating regimen is an eating plan worked out to help individuals experiencing renal infections support the viability of treatment by limiting the degrees of byproducts in their blood.

The renal eating routine is intended to cause as meager additional work or weight on the harmed kidneys as could be expected, while as yet giving adequate great supplements and energy that the body needs.

A renal eating regimen follows a few essential rules. The main rule is that it should be a reasonable, solid, and practical eating regimen, plentiful in filaments, nutrients, regular grains, starches, omega 3 fats, and liquids. Proteins ought to be satisfactory, however not unnecessary.

The salts that are probably going to collect in the circulatory system, are kept to a base. Blood electrolyte levels are checked consistently and the eating regimen changed likewise. It is vital to follow explicit guidance from your PCP and dietitian.

Everyday protein admission is imperative to remake tissues, however ought to be kept to a base. Unnecessary proteins should be separated by the body into carbs and nitrates. Nitrates are not utilized by the body and must be discharged through the kidneys.

Carbs are a significant wellspring of energy and ought to be taken in sufficient amounts. Entire grains and crude types of carbs are awesome. Stay away from profoundly refined starches.

Table salt ought to be limited to cooking as it were. Abundance salt causes liquid maintenance and stresses the kidneys. Pungent nourishments, for example, prepared meats; frankfurters, many tinned food sources, and tidbits ought to be kept away from.

Phosphorus is fundamental for the body to work appropriately, yet dialysis can't eliminate it, so levels should be checked cautiously and admission ought to be restricted however not dispensed with.

Food sources, for example, dairy items, vegetables, and more obscure shaded beverages like colas, have high phosphorus substances. Nourishments high in the potassium content, for example, dim verdant green vegetables, bananas, apricots, and citrus natural products, may likewise be confined if blood levels rise.

Omega 3 fats are a significant piece of any sound eating regimen. Greasy fish is a phenomenal source. Omega fats are fundamental for solid body working. Stay away from trans-fats or hydrolyzed fats.

Liquids ought to be sufficient, yet may be limited in instances of liquid maintenance.

A solid renal eating regimen can help hold kidney work for more. The principle contrasts between any sound eating regimen and a renal eating routine, are the limitations set on protein and table salt admission. Limitations on phosphorus, potassium, and liquids may get essential as side effects and indications of gathering become obvious.

Secrets Of Kidney Disease

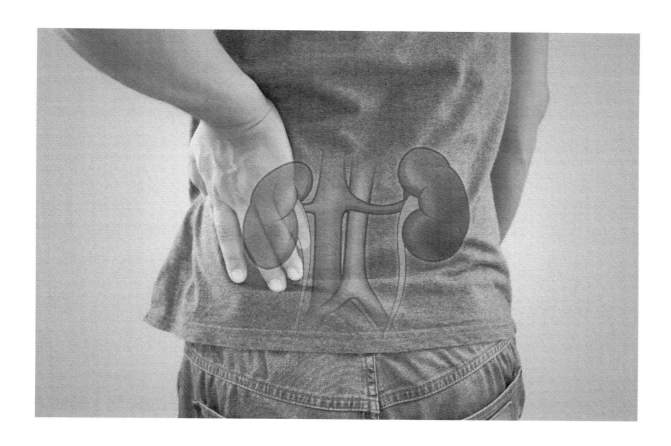

Our kidneys are vital to us. Without effectively working kidneys, the presence of kidney sickness can be wrecking for an individual. In the direst outcome imaginable, an individual should be on dialysis or get a kidney to relocate to supplant the sick kidneys.

There are a few distinct kinds of kidney sickness, some of which are more terrible than others. Kidney infection can be "intense", which means it is of a quick beginning or "constant" which means the decrease in kidney work is moderate. The two sorts of kidney illnesses can be because of immune system issues, poisons, drugs, or diseases. Infections like diabetes and hypertension can step by step demolish the capacity of the kidneys.

Another arrangement of kidney infection happens when the kidneys spill out certain body liquids or substances. One of these sicknesses is hematuria or blood in the pee. This can emerge out of nauseated kidneys that break out platelets from the vessels in the kidneys. The other is genuinely normal and is called proteinuria. Proteinuria is when protein, generally egg whites, spills out from the body. This can turn out to be extraordinary to such an extent that there isn't sufficient protein in the blood of the remainder of the body. We need our protein to keep the liquid in the veins and without it, liquid breaks out into the tissues everywhere on the body. This condition is known as "nephrotic disorder".

The presence of kidney stones is another kidney infection. This can happen when an individual secretes a lot of calcium oxalate into the pee and doesn't drink enough water. Uric corrosive can cause kidney stones too. The calcium oxalate or the uric corrosive develops in the urinary zone of the kidneys and encourages into a stone that, whenever passed, turns out to be exceptionally agonizing. Kidney stones don't fit well in the ureters and they stall out, causing a back of pee and extraordinary agony. Diseases can happen with kidney stones also.

Hypertension can cause kidney illness or, now and again, the drugs that treat (hypertension) can mess the kidney up. Sometimes, an individual has a blockage of one of the two supply routes prompting the kidneys. The kidneys react by delivering vasopressin which causes the circulatory strain to rise strikingly. There are explicit pulse prescriptions that address this issue. Now and again, a medical procedure to address the blockage may be finished.

Persistent pyelonephritis is another kidney illness. This is a condition where contamination seeds into the kidneys (one or both) and causes persistent torment and aggravation in the kidneys. Hematuria can result from this sort of kidney contamination.

There is one essential kidney illness that is dangerous. Renal cell carcinoma is a kind of kidney illness that can happen precipitously.

The malignancy can cause torment or seeping in the zone of the kidneys. A CT sweep of the mid-region can identify this type of kidney sickness. Regularly, if the disease doesn't reach out past the external container of the kidney, the kidney can be taken out and the malignancy is exceptionally treatable.

Kidney sickness can be genetic. There are various uncommon genetic kidney infections that bring about spillage of blood or protein from the kidneys. These illnesses can now and again be overseen medicinally yet, in different cases, dialysis or kidney relocation are important to fix the hidden issue.

Challenge Yourself To Living Healthier In 30 Days!

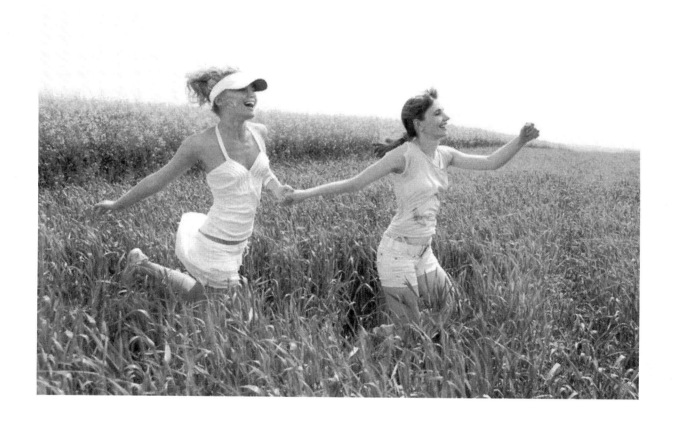

Everybody ought to have an objective of living better. You should need to eat better and to get work out. Studies have indicated that individuals who get fit as a fiddle and stay fit as a fiddle carry on with longer lives, have more energy, and are simply more joyful individuals right around. There are a few things that you can do to challenge yourself in the following 30 days to carry on with a better way of life.

There have been various examinations done that show that a propensity (positive or negative) is framed in 30 days. Indeed, we need to make a decent propensity. In this way, throughout the following month, make a stride in every one of these zones to carry on with a better way of life.

Above all else, in the event that you are not doing anything as of now, you need to begin an activity program. In the event that doesn't need to be untouched burning-through or costly. Something as straightforward as strolling for 15 minutes per day to begin is great. You can run, cycle, in-line skate, sit-ups - anything to get your body going. On the off chance that you have an activity program set up - amazing! How regularly do you work out? One day seven days, two days? Make one of your propensities to practice more. You may need to get up ½ hour sooner - however, the benefits are well justified, despite all the trouble!

Your next propensity is to ensure that you are eating better. This implies eating 5 servings of products of the soil every day. Everybody needs to get this into their eating plans. That numerous servings of leafy foods seem as though parcel - however, is simpler than you might suspect. Also, a simple method to do it is by making smoothies. 5 servings pass by actually rapidly in the event that you put the correct fixings in them!

Another propensity that you need to get into is to ensure that you are drinking 64 ounces of water every day. I realize that there have been some out there now that are saying that this isn't the situation. All things considered, there is an excessive number of clinical specialists who say you ought to. Drinking satisfactory water flushes out the poisons in your body and conveys supplements to your cells. Drinking water additionally assists with keeping our skin and hair sound. We likewise need to keep our bodies hydrated. Lack of hydration can prompt a wide range of issues. Remaining hydrated is additionally significant in light of the fact that you need to renew the liquids that you will lose by perspiring as you work out.

Thus, there you go. That is your test for the following 30 days. Start practicing more, eating better and drinking water each day and perceive how much better you feel!

Am I Suitable For Peritoneal Dialysis?

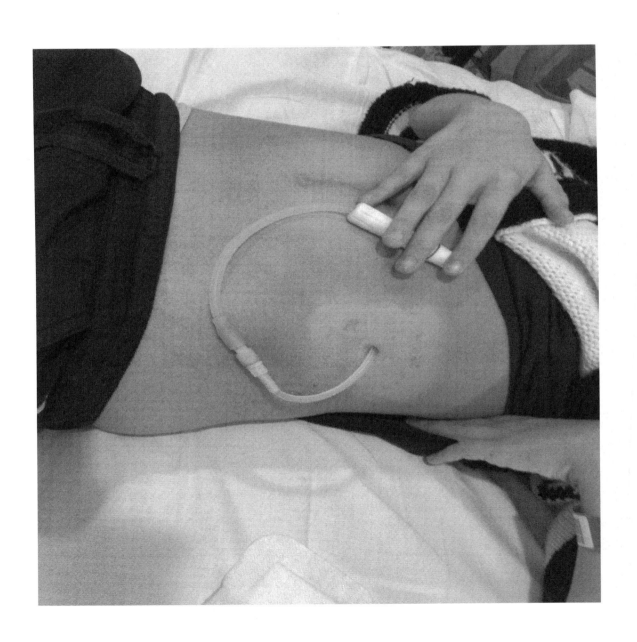

The short answer is very prone to be yes.

Numerous patients find that they are offered hemodialysis by their expert as their first (or here and there their lone) decision. This is conceivably in light of the fact that the expert needs you to be in a controlled climate, which is definitely not something terrible in itself. (Albeit a few people say it is on the grounds that hemodialysis facilities are huge business, as they are supported in the US by the public authority.) The quantity of patients on peritoneal dialysis is unquestionably much lower than those on hemodialysis, and furthermore lower than anticipated dependent on how the medicines work (just one of every ten dialysis patient gets PD treatment).

For some renal disappointment patients, peritoneal dialysis is truth be told a totally practical alternative, and it can let loose them to travel, have occasions, hold down everyday work, and evade customary tedious visits to a kidney center.

However, I've had a transfer and it fizzled!

Indeed, research by a few distinct gatherings of researchers shows that there is no distinction in endurance rates between the individuals who are new PD patients and the individuals who change to PD after a bombed relocation. Nor was there any distinction in the number of patients who figured out how to proceed on the PD program.

However, I'm overweight!

Sadly being fat is getting more normal (particularly among Americans), and as you presumably know, one of the fundamental drivers of kidney disappointment is type 2 diabetes, which likewise causes corpulence. Nonetheless, you do need to be somewhat more cautious on the off chance that you are overweight, as you might be vulnerable to diseases brought about by the catheter, and the danger of peritonitis is higher in the event that you are overweight. One potential arrangement is to utilize a chest catheter (called a presternal catheter). In any case, unfortunately, the more overweight you are, the lower the endurance rate is. More youthful patients with a weight issue have a superior possibility, however, it appears to be that for more established stout patients hemodialysis might be a superior choice.

Be that as it may, I'm somewhat old (in my 80s)!

Without help from anyone else, age ought not to be considered as an obstruction to peritoneal dialysis. Except if you experience the ill effects of shuddering hands or have joint torment, which makes dealing with the PD hardware troublesome, it appears to be that numerous more established patients are very fit for setting up their PD meetings. You do need to have the option to lift the PD sacks notwithstanding, which may make things hard for some old patients living without help from anyone else. Aside from these focuses, don't preclude PD on age alone.

Be that as it may, I've had a hernia!

At that point, you must have it fixed - typically by the lattice treatment under nearby sedation. Furthermore, why not have the passage fitted simultaneously? Exploration shows that this maintenance and fitting cycle is a protected and successful approach to initiate peritoneal dialysis. Also, in the event that you get a hernia subsequent to beginning PD, it doesn't really mean you should change to hemodialysis. It is suggested that on the off chance that you do require a hernia fixed subsequent to beginning PD, you should do your PD meetings resting for half a month thereafter. Doing this decreases the tension on the lines, giving the cross-section a superior possibility of tackling its work and completely fix the hernia.

Be that as it may, I've had peritonitis!

Sadly, this is somewhat all the more a gem. The peritoneal film may have been scarred, precluding PD as an alternative. On the off chance that you get peritonitis during the beginning phases of beginning on PD, you will likely need to change to hemodialysis. So in some cases, PD is conceivable, yet it isn't as regular a choice in these conditions.

However, I'm visually impaired!

Being outwardly weakened makes utilizing a cycler somewhat troublesome, except if somebody concocts one that addresses you. Helpless vision is frequently an issue for those with diabetes, as this is a known result. Then again CAPD is entirely conceivable on the off chance that you are visually impaired, as everything is somewhere around the hand. You may require additional preparation and need to utilize prefilled needles, however, it very well may be finished.

All in all, in the event that you are revealed to you, should take hemodialysis, inquire as to why peritoneal dialysis isn't a choice. Regularly the explanation may very well be "on the grounds that we offer hemodialysis". Ask precisely for what valid reason you by and by can't have PD. It's your decision.

Kidney Cleanse And Its Recipes

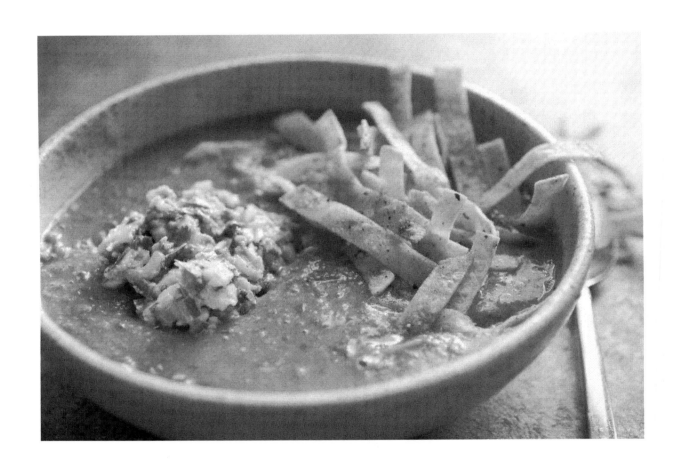

A kidney purge is a technique expected at vanishing kidney stones - stones created inside kidneys. Kidney scrub can likewise be used for recuperating kidney wellbeing by cleaning out poisons developed inside the organ's tissues.

Kidney purify can be so critical, in spite of the fact that you don't encounter lower back torment. There are numerous natural plans, and hundreds of different homeopathic cures used for purifying kidney stones, some of them are:

- Watermelon Cleanse. The simplest approach to do a kidney purify is to get 20 to 100 pounds of watermelon, sit in a shower documented with water, eat as a significant part of the watermelon as possible all as the day progressed, while reliably purging your bladder. This kidney purge isn't fitting for diabetics.

- Celery Seed Tea

- Kidney Cleanse from Dr. Hulda Clark's book, The Cure for All Diseases, clarifies top to bottom how to scrub the kidneys, and her purifying project will dispose of most if not all the stones, without surgery. It is simple or not confounded.

- Corn-silk tea is the incredible single spice for rising pee stream and reestablishing the kidneys.

- Parsley leaves and root tea is for the most part used for kidney purification.

- Parsley seeds are likewise diuretics and are used for separating kidney stones.

- Lemonade diet is a kidney purify to.

- A juice quick is a kidney purify too. Juice fasting (vegetable juices) is used for purging kidneys.

- Treatment of water

It is exceptionally important to purify the kidneys to dispose of the calcium stores and control secret diseases, so keeping away from a sudden breakdown. An individual more than forty ought to totally discover it necessary to do a kidney purify in light of the fact that they are in the most serious danger of a breakdown.

The purifies could be refined all through your typical working week and ought to be done half a month. The upsides of doing a legitimate purify program, be it for colon, liver, kidney or for every one of the three, can be significant.

MALINA PRONTO

Made in the USA
Columbia, SC
08 November 2022